How to engage in unprotected sexual activity without becoming pregnant

Determine your menstrual cycle and identify the safest days for you.

Paul D. Wold

Table of contents

Chapter 1
Chapter 2
Chapter 3

Chapter 1

You should be aware of how to calculate an infertile phase after finding a faithful spouse, as this will enable you to choose when to hit it RAW and prevent getting pregnant.

How quickly can you become pregnant after your period ends?

Pregnancy can only happen if there is sperm in your uterus or fallopian tubes at the time of ovulation. Sperm can remain in your uterus for up to five days following sexual activity.

Ovulation usually happens on day 14 of the cycle for most women. But engaging in unprotected sexual activity during your

period or beyond your anticipated window of fertility, there's no assurance that you won't become pregnant.

Even for women whose cycles are shorter—the average is 28 to 30 days—having sex during your period increases your chance of getting pregnant. You can become pregnant, for instance, if you ovulate early and have sex close to the end of your period. The safest way to avoid getting pregnant is always to use birth control, condoms, or another form of protection.

Continue reading to find out more about avoiding pregnancy by timing your sex and other methods.

THE WAY THAT OVULATION AND

PREGNANCY WORK?

When a developed egg is released from an ovary, ovulation takes place. An egg matures and is discharged into the fallopian tube once a month or so. It then travels to the uterus and fallopian tubes, where sperm are waiting.

After leaving the ovary, an egg is viable for 12 to 24 hours. After having sex, sperm can survive for up to five days. Following fertilization, an egg is implanted, which typically occurs six to twelve days following ovulation.

It's possible to become pregnant right away following your menstruation. That may occur if you are getting close to your reproductive window and have sex towards the end of your cycle. Conversely, nevertheless,

There is little chance of becoming pregnant just before your period.

The likelihood of becoming pregnant is minimal if you watch ovulation and wait 36 to 48 hours following ovulation. The later in the month you are from ovulation, the lower your chances of becoming pregnant.

Your menstrual period will begin and the uterine lining will shed if pregnancy does not develop.

SUCCESS FERTILITY WINDOW

Finding your "optimal" timing to become pregnant might be accomplished by monitoring your reproductive window. If you're not attempting to get pregnant, it can also assist in preventing pregnancy. It may take several months of tracking your monthly cycle to determine your reproductive window while using dependable birth control.

Ways to Monitor Your Fertile WINDOW

You can determine when your fertile window is by using the following procedure.

• Keep track of the day you begin your menstrual cycle and the total number of days in it for a period of eight to twelve months. Keep in mind that the first complete

Day 1 of your menstrual cycle is known as flow day.

• Next, record the number of days that are the longest and the shortest from your

tracking every month.

• Take the duration of your shortest cycle and subtract 18 days to get the first day of your reproductive window. For instance, deduct 18 from 27 and record day 9 if your shortest cycle was 27 day
• Deduct 11 from the length of your longest cycle to determine the final day of your reproductive window. For instance, you would receive day 19 if it lasted 30 days.
• Your fertile window is the period between the shortest and longest day. That would be between days 9 and 19

in the example above. prevent having unprotected children if you're attempting to prevent getting pregnant.

intercourse in those bygone days.

Chapter 2

USE GUIDE FOR A FERTILITY Schedule

Keeping track of your menstrual cycle and knowing when to expect your period each month can be made simple with a fertility calendar. If you wish to become pregnant or avoid getting pregnant, you can also use it to check for fertility indicators. Your most fertile window can be found by performing the relevant calculations with the knowledge of the length of your cycles. During this window, you can either increase or decrease sexual activity based on your family planning goals.

calculating your average

CYCLE DURATION
• Write the first day of your most recent menstrual cycle on the calendar. You can monitor your cycle with a standard calendar. Take note of the initial day of your

The calendar entry for the last menstrual period (LMP) with a number one. This is how you should always record the initial day on the calendar, and then work your way forward from that day.

For instance, if May 15th was the first day of your LMP, enter or type a 1 on that day in the calendar.

It is always the first day of flow, not the first day of spotting, that marks the beginning of your cycle.

TIP: You can download a free fertility tracker app or use a standard paper or digital calendar to monitor your cycle. If you choose to keep a paper or digital calendar, record your cycle by writing or typing on it. If you utilize an app, make sure it has the pertinent cycle-related data entered.

• To find out how long your cycle is, count the days until your next period. This is something you will only be able to accomplish after completing the full cycle. You can count forward from the first day of your LMP to the last day of your cycle. The day before your next menstruation begins is this one.

For instance, you would count from May 15 through June 12 to determine a cycle length of 29 days if your period began on May 15 and your subsequent period began on June 13.

To find the length of your cycle, you won't need to count forward on a calendar if you're using an app to track the days.

• For a minimum of six months, keep a record of your cycles. There could be significant monthly variations in your cycles. Follow them for a minimum of half a year. After completing this, review the history to determine which cycles are the longest and shortest in your

past. After that, calculate the average cycle length by dividing the total number of days by six.

For instance, after six months, if your cycles ranged from 26 to 31 days, your shortest cycle would be 26 days, and your longest would be 31 days.

The average cycle length, rounded to the nearest two, would be 27.8 if the cycles were 26, 28, 28, 26, 28, and 31. This indicates that a 28-day cycle would be the average for you.

• If at all possible, find out when you ovulate. From day 11 to day 21 of your cycle, you can ovulate at any time. Using the reproductive calendar to reach your goals will be simpler if you can determine the day you typically ovulate.

or stop getting pregnant. Keep an eye out for any symptoms indicating you might be ovulating, like:

elevated cervical mucus

Increase in body warmth at resting level Lower cervical posture

Test for positive ovulation prediction

Recognizing Your Fertile

• Take 18 off the total number of days in the shortest cycle you've ever documented. Examine your recorded cycles from the past six to see which one is the shortest.

months. The total number of days in this cycle is then subtracted by 18.

For instance, if your shortest cycle has a total of 27 days, then taking 18 away would result in

You received a score of 9.

To determine your first fertile day, start counting from the first day of the calendar. Then take out your cycle for this month. Determine the first day of your last menstrual cycle (LMP) and proceed forward by the resultant number. The first day is the one you mark.

It's possible that you could get pregnant during that cycle.

In the event that your outcome was 9, for instance, you would record day 9 on your current cycle calendar and proceed forward to that point. In your reproductive window for this cycle, today is the first fertile .

• Take 11 away from your record's longest cycle. To determine the longest cycle you have ever recorded, go back and review your records. The total number of days in this cycle is then subtracted by 11.

If your longest cycle was 32 days in total, for instance, minus 11 would leave you with 21 days.

• Use the calendar to discover the last day that is fertile. Restart your calendar with day 1 and count to

the outcome you get by taking 11 out of your longest cycle. This will provide you with your fertile window's expiration date. Put this day on your schedule.

For instance, if your result was 21, the end of your fertile window for this cycle would be marked on your calendar on day 21.

Chapter 3

Using a fertility calendar to achieve or avoid pregnancy

Engage in sexual activity every day while you are fertile to conceive. Once you are aware of when your periods are,

are, you can ensure that you engage in sexual activity during these times to boost your chances of getting pregnant. If at all possible, engage in sexual activity every other day. However, since eggs remain viable for

12 to 24 hours after release and sperm can survive up to 5 days in the vaginal canal, even every other day of activity may be sufficient to conceive.

For instance, if the days 9 through 21 of your cycle are when you are most fertile, then engage in sexual activity everyday or every other day during this time.

TIP: Using an ovulation predictor kit can help you anticipate ovulation more accurately because you can ovulate at any time between day 11 and day 21 of your cycle. These sets are

extensively accessible over the counter in pharmacies and supermarkets.

To identify your reproductive window, keep an eye on further indicators of fertility. While determining your fertile days can be achieved by using a fertility calendar,

and get pregnant, you might also need to consider other indicators. You can also utilize the following additional indicators to ascertain when you are at your most fertile:

The temperature of the body during rest. Usually, an increase in basal body temperature signifies impending ovulation.

cervical secretions. At your most fertile, cervical mucus has the consistency of egg white.

posture of the cervical region. You will know you are most fertile when your cervix feels low and soft.

DURING YOUR FERTILE WINDOW, USE A CONDOM TO AVOID PREGNANCY

You will need to take extra care during your reproductive window if you intend to avoid getting pregnant and you are not on birth control. Use barrier contraception, such as a condom or diaphragm, or refrain from having intercourse while you are fertile.

Remember that there are circumstances in which it is not advisable to use a fertility calendar to avoid becoming pregnant. For instance, if you are going through menopause, have PCOS, recently gave birth, have an irregular cycle, or have stopped taking birth control, then

You can have erratic cycles.

APPLICATION OF YOUR FERTILE AS A BIRTH CONTROL WINDOW

You will ovulate at some point throughout your reproductive window. The released egg has a 12- to 24-hour viability period. That being said, this window does not allow for daily pregnancy. However, you should avoid having unprotected intercourse for the duration of the fertile window if you're attempting to avoid getting pregnant.

Instruments for monitoring your cycle

Put the first day of your menstrual period on the calendar or in your day planner to keep track of your cycle. Spread out this over a few months. To assist you with keeping track, you can also utilize a fertility app like Clue Period Tracker or Glow Ovulation.

Is the Fertile Approach
SUFFICIENT?

Being aware of your reproductive
window can assist you in avoiding
getting pregnant if your cycles are
extremely regular. Remember, though,
that each month, your cycle days may
still vary. The number of days in your
cycle can vary depending on factors
like stress, nutrition, or intense
exercise. Every month, the day of
ovulation can also vary.

Monitoring your ovulation is a more
successful approach to conceiving.

Discuss the best birth control option with your doctor if you're attempting to avoid getting pregnant.

ADVANCED FERTILITY CONSCIENCE METHODS

Another useful technique for raising awareness of fertility is tracking ovulation. Typical techniques to monitor ovulation include:

monitoring your core body temperature

examining cervical mucus

utilizing kits for ovulation prediction

normal body temperature

The temperature of your body at complete rest is known as your basal body temperature. It rises a little after ovulation. You will require a specialized basal temperature thermometer to monitor your basal body temperature.

Take and note your temperature with the thermometer when you first

get out of bed first thing in the morning. You can use an app or paper to chart it. During ovulation, your body temperature will rise by around 0.5°F (0.3°C).

By delaying unprotected intercourse until a few days following the temperature spike, this strategy is more effective in preventing pregnancy since it enables you to determine when ovulation has happened.

cervical secretions

Near ovulation, some women report an increase in cervical mucus. This is because your cervix produces more mucus during this period due to an increase in estrogen levels.

This mucus will be elastic and transparent. It will have a consistency akin to that of egg whites. On days when you detect a rise in cervical mucus, your body can be most fertile.

kits for predicting ovulation

An ovulation prediction kit can be something you want to get if you're trying to get pregnant. They check for an increase in luteinizing hormone (LH) in your urine.

24 to 48 hours before ovulation, LH increases. Try not to get pregnant at this period by engaging in unprotected sex. However, you would also want to avoid unprotected sex during the five days before this surge, which can be

more difficult to anticipate in advance, because sperm can survive in the uterus for up to five days.

ADDITIONAL FORMATS OF PERCEPTION

Effective contraceptive methods come in a variety of possibilities. Popular options consist of:

birth control tablets

intrauterine gadgets

If you take the recommended precautions, these choices are almost

99 percent successful in preventing pregnancy.

Another reliable method of birth control that offers protection from STDs is the condom.

SUGGESTIONS

The calendar should be hung in a discreet location that is simple to reach, like your bedroom. A carry-around pocket calendar

in your backpack or handbag is an excellent choice as well.

To make it simpler to distinguish between the various phases of your cycle, color-code your fertility calendar. You may, for instance, use a green marker to indicate the days of your cycle when you are unable to conceive, a purple marker to indicate the days of your period, and a red marker to indicate the days of your period.

Cautionary notes

Using a fertility calendar is only advised for partners in monogamous relationships, as unprotected sex can still result in the transmission of a sexually transmitted infection. If you are in many relationships, consider using a barrier form of birth control.

Using a fertility calendar to avoid getting pregnant is not 100% effective! Even with careful monitoring, there is still a possibility that you could become pregnant. See your doctor about different methods of contraception if you believe that you do not want to get pregnant.

FINAL VERDICT

Having unprotected sex when you are menstruating reduces your chances of getting pregnant. It's not a guarantee, though.

Keeping track of ovulation and figuring out when you are fertile will help you reduce your monthly chances of becoming pregnant. The failure rate of natural family planning is approximately 25%. The best course of action if you wish to avoid getting pregnant is to discuss with your doctor a more dependable method of delivery.